Scud Clouds

Scud Clouds

Poems

David Keller and Eloise Bruce

Ragged Sky Press
Princeton, New Jersey

Published by Ragged Sky Press
270 Griggs Drive
Princeton, NJ 08540
www.raggedsky.com

Library of Congress Control Number: 2020934720
ISBN: 978-1-933974-37-8

Cover and book design: Lois Marie Harrod
Photograph of authors: Jim Keller
Cover and interior art: Kevin C. Pyle
Printed in the United States of America
First Edition 2020

Contents

Remember These Three Words

Lesions

Winter and

Foreword

We are poets and for many years we have written
about our life both separately and together. This
book is a result of a journey that began in earnest
when David's Uncle George was diagnosed with a
very rare form of dementia called CADASIL, cerebral
autosomal dominant arteriopathy with subcortical
infarcts and leukoencephalopathy. It is one of those
diseases that run in families: If one parent has it, there
is a 50% chance their child will have it. The trajectory
of the disease was not identified before George
Keller was diagnosed, though it is certain the gene
had been passed down for a very long time. David's
grandmother and his father died in their fifties before
their symptoms presented.

David is in interesting company; it is thought
that the Victorian critic John Ruskin suffered from
CADASIL. Ruskin reported in his diaries having
visual disturbances consistent with the disease, and
it has also been suggested that it might have been a
factor in causing him to describe James Whistler's
Nocturne in Black and Gold — The Falling Rocket as
"ask[ing] two hundred guineas for flinging a pot
of paint in the public's face." The philosopher
Friedrich Nietzsche may have had CADASIL rather
than tertiary syphilis; and both Felix Mendelssohn

and his sister Fanny likely had the disease. Even today it is often misdiagnosed as Parkinson's or MS. Though Willem de Kooning had Alzheimer's and not CADASIL, David was fascinated by a visit to MOMA with Baron and Janet Wormser. He remembers Baron speaking about what he saw as the positive effects of dementia on de Kooning's paintings of that last and late period. David also sees the mysterious ways in which his dementia has shaped his writing since he was diagnosed.

For many the disease is diagnosed in their thirties, but for David's family it presents very late. David was finally diagnosed in 2011, when he was about to turn seventy. The journey toward that diagnosis was not fast or direct. David was having odd symptoms that included passing out, hallucinations, loss of executive function and balance. When he was writing he would sometimes slump over and wake later. Once he was supposed to pick me up at the train station and I waited for several hours, and when I finally arrived home he had covered the floor with pots and pans and had put one piece of dry dog food in each. We began getting late notices because he wasn't paying the bills, and at one point he told me there was no money in the bank to buy groceries. Bills from odd purchases, like a really expensive life-insurance policy, came in the mail. At the time David was working as a carpenter, and he could no longer safely go up a ladder. There were visits to the emergency room, doctors, and many tests that baffled. We were trying to find a neurologist who knew what CADASIL was, much less knowing how to treat it.

In 2011 we finally ended up at the University of Pennsylvania, with a brilliant diagnostician, Murray Grossman, who confirmed that it was CADASIL and pointed us to David Lynch, a specialist in pediatric neurology but who had seen the disease before and had seen it in adults. Finally, David had the blood test that confirmed he had exactly what we thought, a form of dementia that is little understood and has no treatment or cure.

David continues to write, though he has trouble with the computer. He published a book of poetry in 2014. I continue to work part-time as a teaching artist as I have done for many years. We go once a year to visit our current neurologist Dr. Gediminas Gliebus, who always comments on how well we deal with the disease; I think that is largely because David is a very happy person. We also have some support systems that have worked pretty well so far. Like all of us, we live in a house of cards that could tumble at any moment.

We decided to make these poems public because there are so many families being affected by dementia of all kinds, and, having had this experience, we know how difficult it is for people even now to speak about it. We don't intend for this to be a how-to book because that is not the way poetry works. We offer these poems to do what poetry does in all of its elusive and mysterious ways.

—Eloise Bruce

Not

We sing the groan not the giggle.
We dance the ache not the ease
and write the echo not the words,
not the memoir but the glimpse.

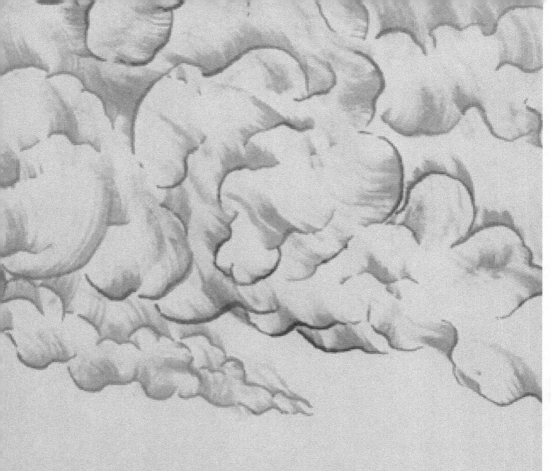

Remember These Three Words

At the Movies

And as the men began swimming for the surface,
I knew what the orange glow above them meant:
fire, oil burning on the sea. You have to be
careful, swimming through the stuff, using
the breaststroke so as to keep the flames
away from you and the death that was certain
if you breathed in the fire.

Strangest of all was that, without thinking,
I knew where I'd learned this:
the year I joined the Boy Scouts, say, sixth grade.
Since none of our leaders knew knots
or anything that might be appealing
and keep us from insurrection, each week
we watched an episode of survival films
courtesy of the US Air Force training.

I still remember how to set a fighter
down in the snow, with its wheels up,
and the consequent wreck if you put down
the gear; or that you can drink from the vines
that grow in the jungle, cut open to reveal
the fresh water inside.

I amaze myself some days with what

I can still remember of song lyrics
heard late at night on the radio,
or how to multiply. War, mostly,
was what we played after school,
as if those games and lessons would save us
much later on in our lives
from age or disease or loss, those enemy snipers.

I Was Right

There we are, at a picnic table in New Hampshire,
and she tells me her husband had Alzheimer's disease.
I question her, saying I, too, have begun
to have memory lapses now and again,
and that I worry. She says, I'll give you
the numbers of some eminent New York doctors,
who will tell you, you are wrong. Call me,

and we parted at the end of the evening
as we do every eight years, on average.

Every year on my birthday, I get
a letter from an old friend, and I
send one on hers. We each worry
when it doesn't
come on time,
that the other has died.
This May I got only a cryptic note, saying
she would write when she had good news.
I wonder what she means.

Looking Gla...

...just fancy calling everything you met "Alice," till one
of them answered!

—Lewis Carroll

When we entered the woods
the names suddenly disappeared,
and kale, bungee cord, hollyho....

Our .....
barked at a ......
perched on a br..., watching
and we tried to remember ....
their......
The Broca's area of our brains
fell fallow and sile.....

On the far side of the wood
my name is Alice and so is his,
even the dog answers to Alice
and the bird seems to be Alice too.
The words of a lifetime suspended
somewhere at the beginning
of the alphabet.

Pocky Blatherer

Last night I dreamed an assignment in second grade,
but when I awoke from a quick nap this afternoon,
I looked at my watch, couldn't tell what time
I'd fallen asleep, in danger of sleeping away
the whole afternoon. So I got up, but dissatisfied
and grumpy. It didn't seem like such a big thing
to remember, but it is. I keep track because it's part
of what's being lost, and I try to keep score. A list
of everything I've lost would help somehow.

Winter is like forgetting all warmth, I've always feared it.
I try to keep it at bay. Fat chance,
not today anyway. The world dances like a tide
fading and returning. "Pocky blatherer"
I shout, like a child, my best insult. It shouts it back.

Marriage in Several Genres

White space

where dementia releases the past
and disappears, whole chapters escaping,
Lake Ohrid gone, and *Carmina Burana*,
forgotten *Symphony No. 5*, Father's face,
Mother's voice and memory
of breakfast or why the door opened.
The flickering of frozen Lake Mendota,
slick of adobe and the blue-cap atop
that college dorm on Holyoke Street
evaporate like the mist this morning
or when we climbed Torr Mor with sheep.

Cinematic remembrances
projected on white expanse,
moving fragments of our young skin,
images of rich food, sweet chocolate,
butter, red meat. Paisley, rumpled sheets,
curls of cigarette smoke after.

Insomnia at 3 a.m.

A momentary pattern of light
travels across the bedroom wall.
Headlights of a pickup truck
or SUV passing in the night. A cat
steals through the bushes and beneath
a cicada nymph feeds on nearby roots.

The driver does not answer to the name Ocean
or Cotton. There is likely no one waiting
in a warm bed in some other bedroom.
The driver must have had a drink
and a look at the sliver of moon.
With feet surely cold and aching,
has she said something she regrets?

My name is not Rain or Precious.
I have not been warm in years and
lie awake, awaiting the next trail of lights.

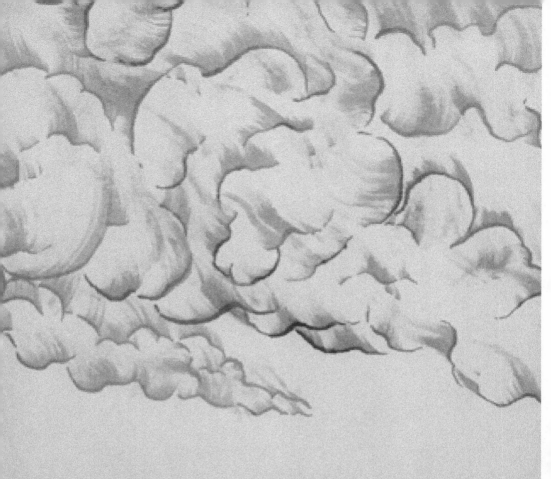

Lesions

And When I Asked Her

The doctor says I have, or will have, dementia,
which I used to think meant something like haunted,
or possessed, like, say, zombies in the comic books;
but it means I will lose my memories, like their teeth.

I hate going to the dentist, a punishment
for not resisting the candy I could never avoid.
Life seems like an old film where you can tell
the good guy by superior dental work.

Not me. Yesterday, sorting through a box of old records,
real vinyl records, on their way to the Goodwill,
I came across a copy of *L'Histoire du soldat*
I must have bought after I heard an old friend

perform it for his Master's recital. Years ago.
But it was a past I didn't know I had forgotten,
and whenever it completely disappears, my friend
who played the percussion part will vanish also.

I suppose. It's odd how we each hope
the coming year will turn out better
than the last one, even though humans know
how things from the past disappear. Not zombies.

To the dentist I must look like one
of the extras in a crowd scene, roaring from pain
and shame, my bad memories.
Oh Doctor K, tell me something different.

100th Love Poem

When we are gone, my love,
rabbits will still breed and rest under our sugi pine.
The bones of our dogs will still rest in its roots
while our nieces and nephews dispose of our paper lanterns
and haul our tansu chests and Nakashima table to the east
and the west, to place them under new eaves.

Children will still walk past
without stopping to gather small pinecones.
Sometimes the little girls will cry
because of some cruelty at school that day.
Miles away the beach and the ocean
would still recognize me and I would speak
words of love to you, I would, if I still had breath.

Snow Days

And I wondered why I mostly include the weather
in my poems. Today, after the snow stopped,
it was like a child who's decided it's been sulking
long enough, so it just stops. It had snowed a foot
during the day, boring, nothing else happening—
no gale winds, no freezing sleet—just snow.
"Dirty Monkey" says Washoe the chimp, learning
to sign. Gradually, I lie down and relax,
and the dog groans, softly.

Last night my wife and I
discussed the list for the grocery shopping,
including a flyer for a special
on pot roast, which she did not think to write down.
But when I'd finished the shopping I could not
remember the last thing I was supposed to get
from the flyer and so didn't buy it.
Oh, to have forgotten a roast so fast.
I'd bought everything on the list and worried
that I was forgetting something, something.
And my wife was distraught and annoyed
one more time. One more not, could not.

"Filthy Monkey" says Washoe, she is learning
to curse. This is how my life proceeds,

nothing systematic, even the way
the mind quits after a long day, going
away. I am sorry, my love, sorry again.
It is not the way I'd expected, again.
I include it so that I may recall how life was:
sad, though not gloomy, a day of melting snow.

Matters of the Heart

My heart aches,
perhaps because I am white and privileged.
I am not equipped to manage a bleeding heart.
But an ache, that I can manage.
I had two sisters, one stillborn and the other aborted
by my divorced mother when I was ten.
Of my two brothers,
one died three years ago,
dropping dead of a heart attack.
He fell face first onto his kitchen floor.
He didn't have time
to reach out his hands to break his fall.
We were fighting at the time
and my own heart aches
that we left it that way in the end.
I ache for my one remaining brother
trapped in his body by schizophrenia.
Diagnosed at fifteen, now he is old
with missing teeth and bad knees.
I ache that my mother only told him
of his illness on her deathbed.
I ache that he had spent a lifetime
of bar brawling and being a mean drunk.
I ache for my husband with his dementia
which has no treatment or cure,

how he loses his balance and stumbles
when he walks, how he
cannot remember the steps of making cookies
unless I read them to him
over and over and how he asks me
what we are having for dinner over and over again.
I am not made to bleed but to ache.
I am filled up with ache
the same way lungs fill with air.
This morning I try to ache for the people
devastated by bombs, famine, earthquakes
and monster storms. I really try
and the ache goes out and the ache comes in.
My ache is involuntary
and I cannot live without it
because it assures me that I am alive.

No Title Comes to Mind

A flutter of pages and leaves
as his poem appears in the *New Yorker* and
her poem is picked by a former poet laureate.
My poems are prisoners in my brain
dulled by the death of our dog,
by the dementia hardening my husband's arteries
and by my old friend imprisoned in her brain by ALS.
What use is recording a world where
the laurel has no bird,
the pages have no numbers,
and the sound of no hand clapping
fills each moment to the fucking brim.

Poem, Beginning "Whatever"

Whatever the usual end of winter
over the past few years
has come to look like or even to mean
for our hearts too easily trampled
by cold and rain, not to mention
gloom-sending winds of Februarys past,
is gone for a while. The air is warm,
and though we are openly glad, we do not
trust ourselves, quite, to this world.
All the nights this week I have dreamed
of dementia and questioned myself to no avail:
will I know when it is here for real, as one might say?

I had been reading an article
on how a dead giraffe in the National Zoo in Copenhagen
was being dissected in public for the sake of knowledge,
while our hero sits wondering
what it would it be like to not know
how to get home after a trip to somewhere
I've gone a million times, or to have an old friend
show up at my door and not recognize his face
until my wife says his name.

Outside, the third of three sunny days in a row
is clouding over for the afternoon,

as expected from the newspaper reports this week.
It's been a good week; one contestant
from the high school recited Frank O'Hara's poem,
"The Day Lady Died," a terrific favorite I'd forgotten
which ends with everyone in the place, and the speaker,
having stopped breathing; I realize that it's a trick
because the speaker is still alive afterwards,
but still the prospect of dying and of dementia
that will preface it is present;
or will it be like forgetting how to brush my teeth.
—I can't grasp that, but it will come to pass.

And here, in the middle of the journey,
I can look up and see, because it has been a long winter
even if not so cold as in other years,
I can look up and see three children down the street
racing back and forth across their yards like starlings.
Having seen their joy, I can look away again.

Sweat

A mile isn't always a mile
as I remember it. That particular one
so long ago, flashes, snaps
and finds its shape
and proper length
in the flex of memory.

I ran away for the first time that summer
with only my short legs to carry me,
wrapped in a blanket of humidity
pulling a red wagon filled
with my stuffed animals and dolls.
The dust rising from the friction
between the wheels and the dirt road
and in a moment I am at the gas station
on the highway drinking a Coca-Cola.

Today I think of running away
and remember what it will take
to walk that actual mile, the dust, dirt and
humidity and having my legs carry me.
I cannot imagine there would be enough room
for everything I love in that little red wagon.

Just the thought fills my lungs with hot,
hot air and it is hard to catch my breath.

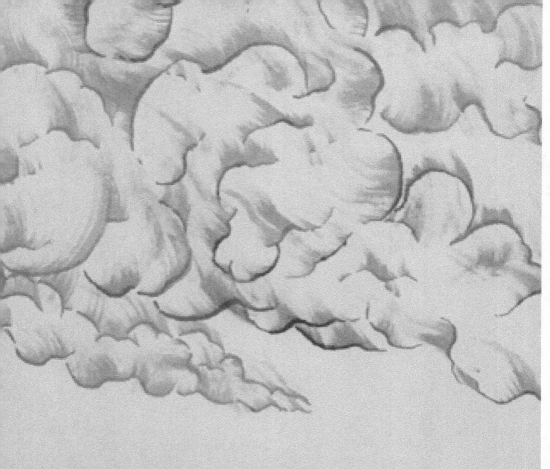

Winter and

October the Second, Like the King

A large chunk of the books I have owned
went out the door this week like heavy
oversized leaves in the rain. And
going through them was like finding
adventures I'd forgotten I had been part of
—a neighbor's dog who had suddenly appeared
on the front porch with no explanation
after being missing for years.

There's always not a lot going on around here,
despite what I say.
Once, when my dog got run over by a car,
I remember I wept for days. He should not
have followed me. After that
only at stories, or watching films of loss.

Perhaps that's why I like owning books.
When Charles Crumb moved to my town, third grade,
and offered to let me help draw
the comic books he created, I was
always cautious, but that didn't help much.
I was never any good at it, though I pretended
well. One day the art teacher pounded Charles's head
on the table; the rage for justice
finally overtook me, and I let her get fired

and said nothing.

For the last two nights
my dreams have been concerned with
forgetting who I am,
unable to find my way home
or to explain why I do not know my name
when asked by the kindly policemen and
someday I may not remember
even your name, your lovely name.

Vertices Intersect

The familiar feel of our fraying cuffs and collars
is only a reminder to avoid things that sparkle
with their glinting sharp edges.
The edges of things make me uneasy.
Arriving at the brink of what we have known.
We have stood at the vast rims of the Sargasso Sea
and Macedonian lakes, the atolls of the South Pacific
and the warm curve of the Gulf Stream. We have peered from
cliffs of Mizen and Malin Head into rolling and boiling seas.

Putting our faith in gravity we practice death in living,
perpetually clinging to the earth at the point where it meets air.
I like to imagine the passing of those I love,
not in gruesome ways but ones that comfort.

I make up stories sometimes with little basis in fact,
awash in blazes of golden light where God
meddles in the affairs of dying. I am a liar
when it comes to death and its ugly foreshadowings.

I want to forget the screams when bowels inflame,
the unimpeded falling face down when hearts stop and
the long plunges from cliff-top onto rock-hard water.

Redefining Crone

Afternoon, June 21—
one layer at a time
I watch my husband's brain
revealed one flat sliver at a time
on the shiny screen
in the doctor's examining room.
The outside edges
of each slice eaten away,
nibbled relentlessly
like Hansel and Gretel
gnawing at the witch's candy house.

Wee hours August 25—
no sleeping beauties here. I am sleepless,
wearing all that is ugly. Past and future
paused in my worn out skull,
or maybe because my bowels are weak and yet not moving,
or my dreams have been invaded by an understanding
that I am always standing on someone else's back.

Every waking moment August 25 thru October 1—
I told myself that I was good
and that if I were good
and tried really hard it would be…
In a letter to my sleepless sisters I will tell them

that goodness makes no difference at all.

Wee hours October 1—
witness to 23,607 moonrises,
husband disappearing.

I Love You

We knew our blood would freeze
and we kept saying *we loved*
and the warm breaths and the soft sounds
seeped into the cracks around the words
until they became a destination
and we hung a hammock
between the *I* and the *You*
so we could rest.

The Surprise

Out of what you'd call a cold snap, or just winter,
without a warning the daffodils bloomed,
the ones called King Alfred, I think,
and everything turned spring-like.
I paused to watch the flowers,
three weeks early. It was
as if this were the end of November, winter
just round the block. And when I looked up again,
the forsythia was beginning already
across the street. Though it had not been

a particularly nasty time; I was glad
to see signs of it leaving,
but it was too fast. The days felt
like a teenager driving a new car
without much control, without
any control. The nameless bushes
in the neighbor's yard were sprouting
green tips on the branch ends,
and patches of reddish light filled the tops
of the trees. Slow down, I thought.

This week I went to an art show opening
where I knew two of the artists,
and everyone standing around drinking

35

wine from plastic glasses was old, seriously
old—grey hair and canes—and I was, too,
as if we were already dead, all.
I will be glad of spring here.

Regret

I might mislead when I describe the contents;
I was asleep when I brought him the box
containing a vial of my blood,
oddly shaped seeds and roots,
a microchip with plans,
various ever-changing cyber chatter,
photos and tintypes of my ancestors
and the bicuspids of an unnamed saint.
There were other items
but I am remembering
and swim in the imperfection of it all.

I did not give these things to him and
still he said, *I must sing an ancient song to know.*
He did and it was long and bored me
so I fell asleep within sleep.

When I woke the box was gone
with him, I assume, to some far place.
There were also grains of sand in the box,
I forgot to tell you that
until I remembered
how I have dreamed so many dreams within dreams.

The Possibility of Silence

From the front, just another of the brownstones
on the block in Philly, but once you enter the long hall
you come to your room, two rooms really,
one that has a large, round bathtub in its center
and, beyond that, the back entrance.
Once there you pass to a yard
almost filled by a picnic table, through another door,
and you've left the house and yard already
for a small street. It's early morning
and you could turn left or right for a walk.
The sun's barely up, though dusty, the light
squeezed dry, the row of small shops and a tree,
also dust-covered, are deserted.
You seek nothing here but a breath of the daylight
before you leave for the lecture you've come for.
That's hours away, after breakfast, a couple of stale Danish
and a cup of coffee from a mug left on the table. No grapes.

You hardly know how close you are to the day's center
in the dream you will have of this in the future
or the evening that led here after a long day's work, here
being a Cuban restaurant and a table for you both outside.
Everything has taken an oath of happiness. Have
another glass of wine, as fall begins once more.
It's only a short trip to your car from the table, and to bed.

Nothing in this dream will make a difference
when you leave. You are grateful for it all
and the laughter. Even for the bathtub you couldn't
figure how to empty and so left full of water.
There is nothing to regret. It will not be filled with pain,
or not for long. Leave laughing. Goodbye.

The Poet Speaks from the Grave

A shoreline is always something unfinished, slipping
away, drifting. A piece of fiction relates to reality in the
same way.

—Henning Mankell

She says there is no frigate
and my husband hunches over
a book on this winter weekday.
He is far away inhabiting
the protagonist whose house
has burned to the ground.
Like that old man, he remembers
places traveled. For my husband
a summer picnic in Macedonia
where gypsies play violins and a cimbalom
on the banks of Lake Ohrid.
Both old men dream
of their childhood. One
of his fictional archipelago, one
of the Anasazi, far above him
gazing down at him from desert cliffs
in the shadow of a mushroom cloud.

My husband grew up far from the sea.
These two old men, one imagined,
the other flesh, are vessels in a sea

of loneliness. They float in it
and are filled up with it.
Today it is an ice-filled Baltic Sea
which cracks, moans,
grumbles, intones like
the pipes of an organ
building to a climax.
The novel my husband devours
is about death,
old men perched on its edge
have a need to navigate its waters
while the shoreline shifts and recedes.

Acknowledgments

Acknowledgment is gratefully made to the editors of the following, where versions of these poems first appeared:

Poem, Beginning "Whatever," *US 1 Worksheets*, 2016.
Regret, *SleepyHead Central*, 2017.
At the Movies, *Spank the Carp*, 2018.

We thank our poetry groups who offered feedback on the poems in the book. We especially thank Cool Women's Lois Marie Harrod for assembling this book and making it look beautiful, and Betty Bonham Lies for being our first reader. We are very grateful to Ragged Sky Press and to publisher Ellen Foos for seeing the value in the book and carefully nurturing it into final form. We thank Kevin Pyle for the cover art and Jim Keller for the photograph of us on the back cover.

Notes

At some point after the diagnosis, I began to include examples of my memory loss in my poems, to record for the future, a kind of keeping score; especially since CADASIL is not like what I know about Alzheimer's. In another example, when a urologist asked me how many times I get up at night to urinate, I realized I could not remember if there had ever been a time when I could sleep through an entire night without getting up.

The piece referred to in the poem "And When I Asked Her" is Igor Stravinsky's *L'Histoire du soldat*.

The entire manuscript owes a debt to *Monty Python and the Holy Grail*, especially the scene called "I Think I'll Go for a Walk."

—David Keller

About the Authors

David Keller was born in Berkeley, California, where his father was finishing work on a PhD. He was raised in Los Alamos, New Mexico, and Ames, Iowa. He was educated at Harvard College and the University of Wisconsin, Madison. The author of five collections of poetry, he has taught poetry workshops in New York City and has served as Assistant Poetry Coordinator for the Geraldine R. Dodge Poetry Festival, on the Board of Governors of the Poetry Society of America, and as a member of the Advisory Board of the Frost Place.

Eloise Bruce was born in Opelika, Alabama, and raised on Anna Maria Island, Florida, and educated at Wesleyan College and Mercer University in Macon, Georgia, and the University of Alabama at Tuscaloosa. She has been an integral part of the planning, implementation and adjudication of Poetry Out Loud in New Jersey since its inception. In 2004 her first book of poetry, *Rattle*, was published by CavanKerry Press. She is a member of the poetry critique and performance group Cool Women. She is the founder of Idaho Theater for Youth and the Youth Editor of *Raven Perch* magazine. Eloise and David met on Christmas

Eve, 1987, in Summertown, a suburb of Oxford, England, and maintained a friendship until 1989, when they fell in love and moved to Lawrenceville, New Jersey, where they still reside. In 1994 they married in Robert Frost's Barn in Franconia, New Hampshire.